Sleep Evolution

Transform Your Life With Revolutionary Sleep Optimization Strategies

Dewey M. Stewart

Table Of Contents

Introduction: Welcome To The Sleep Evolution

In a world that is constantly on the move, where the demands of daily life seem to stretch beyond the limits of time and space, sleep often becomes the silent casualty. The relentless pursuit of success, productivity, and a perpetual sense of urgency has led many to sacrifice the one thing that is foundational to our well-being: quality sleep. However, what if the key to unlocking our fullest potential and transforming our lives lay not in the hours we spend awake, but in the quality of our sleep?

Welcome to "Sleep Evolution: Transform Your Life with Revolutionary Sleep Optimization Strategies." This book is your guide to understanding, harnessing, and mastering the science of sleep. Here, we will explore the depths of how sleep works, why it is crucial, and most importantly, how you can evolve your sleep habits to enhance every aspect of your life.

Embracing Change: Transforming Your Life Through Better Sleep

The concept of evolution is about progress and adaptation. Just as species evolve over time to become better suited to their environments, so too can we evolve our approach to sleep to better suit the modern world. In this book, we invite you to embark on a transformative journey. This is not just about getting more sleep—it's about getting better sleep, and in doing so, transforming your life in ways you may have never thought possible.

Many of us have grown accustomed to the notion that sleep is a passive activity, something that simply happens to us at the end of a long day. However, sleep is an active, dynamic process that plays a critical role in our health, cognitive function, emotional well-being, and overall quality of life. By understanding and optimizing this process, we can unlock a wealth of benefits that extend far beyond the bedroom.

The Modern Sleep Crisis

We are in the midst of a modern sleep crisis. Studies show that a significant portion of the global population is chronically sleep-deprived, and this deprivation is taking a toll on our health and well-being. According to the Centers for Disease Control and Prevention (CDC), more than a third of American adults are not getting the recommended seven or more hours of sleep per night. This epidemic of insufficient sleep is linked to a host of health problems, including obesity, heart disease, diabetes, and mental health disorders such as depression and anxiety.

The consequences of poor sleep are far-reaching and profound. Beyond the immediate effects of fatigue and irritability, chronic sleep deprivation impairs our cognitive function, reducing our ability to concentrate, make decisions, and solve problems. It weakens our immune system, making us more susceptible to illness, and it undermines our emotional resilience, increasing our vulnerability to stress and mood disorders. In short, the quality of our sleep is directly linked to the quality of our lives.

A Revolutionary Approach to Sleep Optimization

In "Sleep Evolution," we will delve into a revolutionary approach to sleep optimization. This approach is rooted in the latest scientific research and draws on a wealth of knowledge from fields such as neuroscience, psychology, and chronobiology. We will explore cutting-edge techniques and strategies that go beyond conventional sleep advice, offering you practical tools and insights to transform your sleep habits and, by extension, your life.

Our journey begins with an in-depth understanding of the science of sleep. By demystifying the complexities of sleep cycles, circadian rhythms, and the biological processes that govern our sleep-wake patterns, we will lay the foundation for effective sleep optimization. Armed with this knowledge, you will be better equipped to make informed decisions about your sleep habits and create a personalized sleep plan that works for you.

Beyond Quantity: The Quality of Sleep

While the quantity of sleep is important, it is the quality of sleep that truly matters. Many of us may get the recommended number of hours of sleep but still wake up feeling tired and unrefreshed. This is because the quality of our sleep can be compromised by various factors, such as stress, poor sleep environment, and unhealthy habits. In this book, we will focus on enhancing the quality of your sleep, ensuring that each hour of rest is restorative and rejuvenating.

We will explore how to create a sleep-friendly environment that promotes deep, restful sleep. From optimizing your bedroom setup to managing light, noise, and temperature, we will provide you with practical tips to transform your sleeping space into a sanctuary of rest and relaxation. We will also delve into the importance of establishing healthy sleep habits and rituals that signal to your body and mind that it is time to wind down and prepare for sleep.

Chapter 1: Understanding Your Sleep Blueprint

Understanding your sleep blueprint is the cornerstone of optimizing your sleep for better health and well-being. Just as a blueprint provides detailed plans for a building, your sleep blueprint offers a comprehensive understanding of the unique patterns, preferences, and needs that define your sleep. By exploring the stages of sleep, circadian rhythms, and individual differences, you can tailor your sleep habits to better suit your needs and improve your overall quality of life.

The Science of Sleep: Stages and Cycles

Sleep is a complex, dynamic process consisting of multiple stages that cycle throughout the night. Each stage plays a crucial role in maintaining our physical and mental health. Understanding these stages can help you appreciate the intricacy of sleep and why it is important to achieve a full night's rest.

There are two main types of sleep: non-rapid eye movement (NREM) sleep and rapid eye movement (REM) sleep. NREM sleep is subdivided into three distinct stages:

1. **Stage 1 (N1):** This is the lightest stage of sleep, lasting only a few minutes. During this stage, you transition from wakefulness to sleep, and your body starts to relax. You may experience sudden muscle jerks or the sensation of falling.

2. **Stage 2 (N2):** This stage constitutes the largest portion of our sleep. It is characterized by a further decrease in muscle activity and a slowing of the heart rate. Brain activity shows distinct patterns, including sleep spindles and K-complexes, which are thought to play a role in memory consolidation and sensory processing.

3. **Stage 3 (N3):** Also known as deep sleep or slow-wave sleep, this stage is crucial for physical restoration and recovery. During deep sleep, the body repairs tissues, builds muscle and bone, and strengthens the immune system. Brain

activity during this stage shows slow, high-amplitude waves known as delta waves.

REM sleep, the fourth stage, is when most dreaming occurs. This stage is characterized by rapid eye movements, increased brain activity, and temporary paralysis of major muscle groups. REM sleep is crucial for cognitive functions like learning, memory, and emotional regulation. The brain processes and consolidates information from the day, and neural connections are strengthened.

A typical night's sleep consists of multiple cycles through these stages, each lasting about 90 minutes. As the night progresses, the proportion of REM sleep increases while deep sleep stages become shorter. Disruptions to this cycle, such as waking up frequently or not getting enough sleep, can impair the restorative functions of sleep and leave you feeling tired and unrefreshed.

Understanding Your Circadian Rhythm

Circadian rhythms are internal biological clocks that regulate the sleep-wake cycle and other physiological processes. They are influenced by external cues such as light and temperature but are also shaped by genetic factors. Your circadian rhythm determines when you feel sleepy and when you are most alert.

Chronotypes are classifications of individual circadian preferences. People are generally categorized as morning types (larks), evening types (owls), or intermediate types. Understanding your chronotype can help you align your activities and sleep schedule with your natural tendencies, making it easier to fall asleep and wake up feeling refreshed.

For instance, if you are a night owl, you may find it challenging to adhere to a traditional 9-to-5 schedule. Conversely, morning larks may struggle with late-night activities. By recognizing your chronotype, you can adjust your schedule to match your natural rhythm, optimizing your performance and well-being.

Identifying Individual Sleep Needs

While the average adult needs about 7-9 hours of sleep per night, individual sleep needs can vary. Factors such as age, lifestyle, and health status influence how much sleep you require. Observe your daytime feelings to assess whether you are getting sufficient sleep. If you feel alert and productive, you are likely meeting your sleep needs. If you experience fatigue, irritability, or difficulty concentrating, you may need to adjust your sleep habits.

To identify your optimal sleep duration, consider conducting a sleep experiment. For a week, allow yourself to sleep without setting an alarm. Track the amount of sleep you get each night and how you feel during the day. This experiment can help you determine the amount of sleep your body naturally requires.

Decoding Your Personal Sleep Patterns and Preferences

Understanding your personal sleep patterns and preferences is a critical step in optimizing your overall health and well-being. Sleep is not a uniform experience for everyone; it varies significantly from person to person, influenced by factors such as genetics, lifestyle, and environmental conditions. By decoding your unique sleep blueprint, you can tailor your habits and environment to better suit your needs, leading to more restful and restorative sleep.

Recognizing Your Sleep Chronotype

One of the fundamental aspects of personal sleep patterns is your sleep chronotype, which refers to your natural inclination for sleeping and waking times. People generally fall into one of three broad categories: morning types (larks), evening types (owls), and intermediate types (hummingbirds).

Morning Types (Larks): These individuals feel most energetic and alert in the early part of the day. They tend to wake up early, often without the need for an alarm, and prefer to go to bed early in the evening. Morning types may find it easier to adapt to traditional work schedules that start early in the day.

Evening Types (Owls): These individuals are most alert and productive in the late afternoon or evening. They often struggle with early mornings and prefer to stay up late. Evening types may find it challenging to adhere to conventional work schedules but can thrive in environments that allow for later start times.

Intermediate Types (Hummingbirds): These individuals have a more flexible sleep-wake pattern and can adjust relatively easily to different schedules. They may not have a strong preference for either morning or evening and can adapt to a variety of routines.

To identify your chronotype, pay attention to your natural tendencies and energy levels throughout the day. Consider keeping a sleep diary for a few weeks, noting the times you feel most awake and alert, as well as when you naturally feel sleepy. This can help you determine your chronotype and align your daily activities accordingly.

Understanding Your Sleep Needs

The amount of sleep each person needs can vary widely. While the average adult requires about 7-9 hours of sleep per night, individual sleep needs depend on various factors, including age, lifestyle, and overall health.

Age: Sleep needs change throughout the lifespan. Newborns and infants require the most sleep, often up to 16-18 hours per day. As children grow, their sleep needs gradually decrease, with teenagers needing about 8-10 hours of sleep per night. Adults typically need 7-9 hours, while older adults may find they need slightly less sleep, often around 7-8 hours.

Lifestyle: Your daily activities and lifestyle choices can significantly impact your sleep needs. High levels of physical activity may increase your need for sleep, as your body requires more time to recover and repair. Stressful or demanding mental tasks can also lead to an increased need for rest and recovery.

Health: Overall health and well-being play a crucial role in determining sleep needs. Conditions such as chronic pain, anxiety, or depression can affect sleep quality and duration. Additionally, sleep disorders like insomnia, sleep apnea, or restless leg syndrome can disrupt normal sleep patterns, leading to increased fatigue and a greater need for rest.

Unveiling the Blueprint for Optimal Sleep Health

Achieving optimal sleep health is a multifaceted process that requires an understanding of the intricate components of sleep and how they interact with your individual lifestyle and needs. The blueprint for optimal sleep health is not a one-size-fits-all approach; it is personalized and adaptable, taking into account your unique sleep patterns, environmental factors, and daily habits. By following a structured plan that encompasses these elements, you can significantly improve the quality of your sleep and, consequently, your overall health and well-being.

Recognizing Individual Differences

The first step in creating a blueprint for optimal sleep health is recognizing that individual differences play a crucial role in sleep. These differences can be broadly categorized into chronotypes, sleep needs, and personal health factors.

Chronotypes: Your chronotype is your natural propensity for sleep and wake times, often classified into morning types (larks), evening types (owls), and intermediate types (hummingbirds). Knowing your chronotype can help you align your sleep schedule with your biological clock, making it easier to fall asleep and wake up feeling refreshed. For instance, morning types might thrive with early bedtimes and wake-up times, while evening types might perform better with later schedules.

Sleep Needs: While the average adult requires 7-9 hours of sleep per night, individual sleep needs can vary. Factors such as age, physical activity, and health status influence how much sleep you need. Adolescents and young adults typically need more sleep than older adults. Listening to your body and paying attention to how you feel during the day can help you determine if you are meeting your sleep needs. Persistent feelings of fatigue or difficulty concentrating may indicate a need for more sleep.

Optimizing Your Sleep Environment

Creating a sleep-friendly environment is essential for promoting restful sleep. This involves controlling light, temperature, and noise levels in your bedroom, as well as ensuring your bed is comfortable.

Light and Darkness: Exposure to natural light during the day helps regulate your circadian rhythm, promoting alertness during waking hours and sleepiness at night. At bedtime, your bedroom should be as dark as possible. Use blackout curtains or a sleep mask to block out light. Reducing exposure to blue light from screens at least an hour before bed can also help facilitate sleep.

Temperature: The optimal temperature for sleep is generally cool, between 60-67°F (15-19°C). A cooler room helps your body lower its core temperature, which is necessary for initiating sleep. Adjust your bedding and sleepwear to maintain comfort throughout the night.

Noise Control: Maintaining a quiet environment is essential for uninterrupted sleep. You may want to use earplugs or a white noise machine to mask disruptive noises. White noise can create a consistent auditory environment that helps you fall asleep faster and stay asleep longer.

Comfort: Invest in a high-quality mattress and pillows that suit your sleep position and comfort preferences. Proper support can prevent discomfort and pain, allowing you to sleep more soundly.

Establishing Healthy Sleep Habits

Healthy sleep habits, often referred to as sleep hygiene, are behaviors that can improve your sleep quality. These include maintaining a consistent sleep schedule, developing a pre-sleep routine, and managing your intake of food and beverages.

Consistent Sleep Schedule: Going to bed and waking up at the same time every day, including weekends, helps regulate your body's internal clock. Consistency reinforces your sleep-wake cycle, making it easier to fall asleep and wake up naturally.

Pre-Sleep Routine: Establish a relaxing pre-sleep routine to signal to your body that it is time to wind down. Engaging in activities like reading, taking a warm bath, or practicing relaxation techniques such as deep breathing or meditation can help prepare your mind and body for sleep.

Food and Beverage Management: Avoid consuming large meals, caffeine, and alcohol close to bedtime. Caffeine and alcohol can interfere with your ability to fall asleep and stay asleep, while heavy meals can cause discomfort and indigestion.

Chapter 2: The Science Of Sleep Transformation

Sleep transformation is a profound journey that involves improving the quality and patterns of sleep through a scientific understanding of sleep processes. This approach goes beyond merely getting enough hours of rest; it delves into optimizing the intricate details of how and why we sleep, considering individual variations and implementing practices based on scientific research to achieve the best possible sleep health.

The Fundamentals of Sleep

To transform sleep effectively, it's crucial to understand the fundamentals of how sleep works. Sleep is composed of two main types: Non-Rapid Eye Movement (NREM) and Rapid Eye Movement (REM) sleep. These types of sleep cycle multiple times throughout the night, each serving essential functions for physical and mental health.

NREM Sleep: NREM sleep consists of three stages, each deeper than the last. The first stage is light sleep, where you transition from wakefulness to sleep. The second stage involves a further slowing of brain waves and body functions, while the third stage, known as deep sleep, is crucial for physical restoration, immune function, and energy recovery.

REM Sleep: During REM sleep, brain activity increases, and vivid dreams occur. REM sleep is essential for cognitive functions, including memory consolidation, learning, and emotional regulation. The alternating cycles of NREM and REM sleep allow the body and mind to rejuvenate and prepare for the next day.

The Role of Circadian Rhythms

Circadian rhythms are the internal clocks that regulate sleep-wake cycles over a 24-hour period. These rhythms are influenced by external cues like light and temperature but are also genetically programmed.

Light Exposure: Natural light helps regulate circadian rhythms by signaling to the brain when it's time to wake up and when it's time to sleep. Exposure to daylight in the morning can help set your internal clock, making it easier to fall asleep at night.

Chronotypes: People have different chronotypes, meaning their natural predisposition for sleeping and waking times varies. Understanding whether you are a morning type (lark), evening type (owl), or somewhere in between can help you schedule activities in alignment with your biological clock, enhancing your productivity and sleep quality.

Lifestyle Factors and Sleep Quality

Lifestyle choices significantly impact sleep quality. Several key habits can either enhance or disrupt your sleep.

Exercise: Engaging in regular physical activity can help you fall asleep more quickly and experience deeper sleep. However, exercising too close to bedtime may have the opposite effect, as it can increase alertness and body temperature.

Diet: What you eat and drink affects sleep. Consuming large meals, caffeine, or alcohol close to bedtime can disrupt sleep. Instead, opt for a light snack if you're hungry before bed and limit stimulants in the hours leading up to sleep.

Routine: Establishing a consistent sleep routine helps signal to your body when it's time to wind down. Going to bed and waking up at the same time every day, even on weekends, can strengthen your body's internal clock.

The Revolutionary Insights: Cutting-Edge Research And Discoveries

In recent years, the field of sleep science has seen groundbreaking advancements that have revolutionized our understanding of sleep and its profound impact on health. Cutting-edge research has unveiled new insights into the mechanisms of sleep, the genetic factors influencing sleep patterns, and the links between sleep and various health outcomes. These discoveries are paving the way for innovative approaches to sleep disorders and personalized sleep medicine.

Genetic Insights into Sleep

One of the most exciting areas of sleep research is the exploration of genetic factors that influence sleep patterns and behaviors. Scientists have identified specific genes that play crucial roles in regulating sleep-wake cycles, circadian rhythms, and sleep duration. For instance, variations in the PER3 gene have been associated with differences in sleep preferences, such as being a morning person or a night owl. Understanding these genetic influences allows for a more personalized approach to managing sleep issues, as interventions can be tailored to an individual's genetic profile.

The Role of Sleep in Brain Function and Neuroplasticity

Recent studies have highlighted the critical role of sleep in brain function and neuroplasticity—the brain's ability to adapt and reorganize itself. During sleep, particularly during REM sleep, the brain processes and consolidates memories, enhances learning, and clears out neurotoxic waste products through the glymphatic system. This system, a network of channels that clear waste from the brain, is most active during sleep, suggesting that sleep is essential for maintaining cognitive health and preventing neurodegenerative diseases such as Alzheimer's.

Sleep and Immune Function

Cutting-edge research has also shed light on the intricate relationship between sleep and the immune system. Sleep is vital for the production and release of cytokines, proteins that help regulate the immune response. Research has demonstrated that lack of sleep can weaken the immune system, increasing susceptibility to infections and illnesses. Conversely, adequate sleep enhances the body's ability to fight off pathogens and recover from illness, highlighting the importance of sleep for overall health and resilience.

The Impact of Technology on Sleep

The advent of digital technology has had a significant impact on sleep patterns, prompting researchers to investigate its effects on sleep quality. Exposure to blue light from screens can suppress the production of melatonin, the hormone that regulates sleep-wake cycles, leading to difficulties in falling asleep. Additionally, the constant connectivity and information overload associated with technology use can contribute to stress and anxiety, further disrupting sleep. Researchers are exploring interventions such as blue light filters, screen time limits, and digital detoxes to mitigate these effects and promote healthy sleep habits.

Sleep and Mental Health

The bidirectional relationship between sleep and mental health is another area of cutting-edge research. Poor sleep is both a symptom and a contributing factor to various mental health disorders, including depression, anxiety, and bipolar disorder. Innovative studies are examining how improving sleep can alleviate symptoms of these conditions and enhance overall mental well-being. Cognitive Behavioral Therapy for Insomnia (CBT-I) is emerging as a highly effective treatment, not only for sleep disorders but also for improving mental health outcomes.

Chronotherapy and Circadian Medicine

Chronotherapy and circadian medicine are rapidly growing fields that focus on aligning medical treatments with the body's natural rhythms. Researchers are investigating how the timing of sleep, meals, medication, and other daily activities can influence health outcomes. For example, studies have shown that aligning chemotherapy treatments with the patient's circadian rhythms can improve efficacy and reduce side effects. This approach underscores the importance of timing in health and disease management, offering new avenues for optimizing treatments and interventions.

Wearable Technology and Sleep Tracking

The development of wearable technology and advanced sleep tracking devices has revolutionized the way we monitor and understand sleep. These devices provide detailed data on sleep stages, heart rate, and movement, offering valuable insights into sleep patterns and potential disturbances. Researchers are leveraging this data to identify trends and correlations that can inform personalized sleep interventions. The integration of artificial intelligence and machine learning with sleep tracking technology is poised to further enhance our understanding of sleep and its implications for health.

The Future of Sleep Medicine

The future of sleep medicine is promising, with ongoing research and technological advancements paving the way for more effective and personalized treatments. From genetic testing to tailor sleep interventions to wearable devices that provide real-time feedback, the field is moving towards a more comprehensive and individualized approach to sleep health. These advancements hold the potential to significantly improve the quality of life for individuals with sleep disorders and to enhance overall public health.

Redefining Sleep Success: Beyond Quantity To Quality

The quest for optimal health and well-being has long emphasized the importance of sleep, traditionally measured in terms of quantity. However, emerging research and evolving perspectives in sleep science have shifted the focus towards the quality of sleep, suggesting that how well we sleep may be as crucial as how long we sleep. Redefining sleep success means moving beyond the simplistic view of counting hours to a more nuanced understanding of the various factors that contribute to restorative and effective sleep.

The Essence of Sleep Quality

Sleep quality encompasses several dimensions: sleep latency (the time it takes to fall asleep), sleep continuity (the absence of frequent awakenings), sleep depth (the extent of deep, restorative sleep), and subjective sleep satisfaction (how rested one feels upon waking). High-quality sleep ensures that an individual cycles adequately through all sleep stages, including light sleep, deep sleep, and REM sleep. Each stage plays a critical role in physical recovery, cognitive processing, and emotional regulation.

Key Determinants of Sleep Quality

1. Sleep Environment: The conditions of the sleep environment are fundamental to achieving high-quality sleep. A bedroom that is cool, quiet, and dark fosters an atmosphere conducive to uninterrupted rest. Noise-canceling devices, blackout curtains, and a comfortable mattress and pillows can enhance the sleep environment significantly. Additionally, limiting exposure to screens and blue light before bedtime helps maintain the natural production of melatonin, the hormone responsible for regulating sleep-wake cycles.

2. Sleep Hygiene: Good sleep hygiene practices are crucial for fostering better sleep quality. This involves maintaining a consistent sleep schedule, even on weekends, to regulate the body's internal clock. Avoiding heavy meals, caffeine, and alcohol close to bedtime can prevent disruptions in sleep patterns. Establishing a relaxing pre-sleep routine, such as reading a book, taking a warm bath, or engaging in light stretching, signals the body that it is time to wind down and prepare for sleep.

3. Mental Health and Stress Management: Stress and anxiety are significant disruptors of sleep quality. High levels of stress can increase the time it takes to fall asleep and lead to frequent awakenings throughout the night. Incorporating relaxation techniques such as mindfulness, meditation, and deep breathing exercises can help calm the mind and prepare the body for restful sleep. Cognitive Behavioral Therapy for Insomnia (CBT-I) has also proven effective for individuals with chronic sleep problems, addressing negative thoughts and behaviors related to sleep.

4. Physical Activity: Regular physical activity is beneficial for sleep quality, as it helps to reduce stress and promote physical tiredness, which can facilitate easier and deeper sleep. However, timing is important; engaging in vigorous exercise too close to bedtime can increase alertness and body temperature, making it harder to fall asleep. Morning or early afternoon workouts are generally more conducive to promoting better sleep at night.

Measuring and Improving Sleep Quality

Advances in technology have made it easier to measure and monitor sleep quality. Wearable devices and sleep-tracking apps provide detailed data on various sleep metrics, including the duration of different sleep stages, sleep interruptions, and overall sleep efficiency. This information can be invaluable for identifying patterns and pinpointing areas for improvement.

1. Sleep Diaries: Keeping a sleep diary can help track sleep habits and identify factors that may be affecting sleep quality. Recording bedtimes, wake times, and any awakenings during the night, along with notes on daily activities, diet, and stress levels, can provide insights into patterns and potential triggers for poor sleep.

2. Personalized Interventions: Based on data from sleep tracking and diaries, personalized interventions can be developed to enhance sleep quality. These may include adjusting sleep schedules, improving sleep environments, or implementing relaxation techniques. Personalized sleep plans can address individual needs and preferences, leading to more effective and sustainable improvements in sleep quality.

The Benefits of High-Quality Sleep

1. Cognitive Function: High-quality sleep is essential for cognitive processes such as memory consolidation, learning, and decision-making. During sleep, the brain processes and stores information from the day, which is crucial for long-term memory and cognitive performance.

2. Physical Health: Quality sleep supports physical health by aiding in the repair and growth of tissues, muscle recovery, and immune function. Deep sleep, in particular, plays a significant role in maintaining physiological systems and promoting overall health.

3. Emotional Well-being: Emotional stability and mental health are closely linked to sleep quality. Poor sleep can lead to increased irritability, mood swings, and a higher risk of mental health disorders such as depression and anxiety. Consistently good sleep helps stabilize emotions and improve overall mental health.

4. Daily Performance: Individuals who consistently achieve high-quality sleep are more alert, focused, and productive during the day. Good sleep quality enhances energy levels, motivation, and the ability to perform daily tasks efficiently.

Chapter 3: Navigating The Inner Landscape: Mind, Body, And Sleep

The intricate relationship between the mind, body, and sleep forms a complex and dynamic triad that profoundly impacts our overall well-being. Understanding and navigating this inner landscape is crucial for optimizing health and enhancing the quality of life. This exploration delves into the interconnectedness of psychological states, physiological processes, and sleep, revealing how each component influences and is influenced by the others.

The Mind and Sleep

The mind plays a pivotal role in the regulation of sleep. Psychological factors such as stress, anxiety, and depression can significantly affect sleep quality and patterns. When the mind is preoccupied with worries or distress, it becomes challenging to relax and fall asleep. This is because the brain's heightened state of alertness interferes with the natural transition into sleep. Chronic stress activates the body's fight-or-flight response, leading to increased levels of cortisol, a hormone that disrupts the sleep-wake cycle.

Mindfulness and relaxation techniques can help mitigate these effects. Practices such as meditation, deep breathing, and progressive muscle relaxation can calm the mind, reduce stress levels, and promote a smoother transition into sleep. Cognitive Behavioral Therapy for Insomnia (CBT-I) is another effective approach, helping individuals reframe negative thoughts about sleep and develop healthy sleep habits.

The Body and Sleep

Physiological processes within the body are equally crucial in determining sleep quality. The body's circadian rhythm, an internal biological clock, regulates the sleep-wake cycle by responding to external cues like light and temperature. This rhythm dictates when we feel awake and when we feel sleepy. Disruptions to this rhythm, such as those caused by irregular sleep schedules, jet lag, or shift work, can lead to sleep disturbances.

Physical health conditions also play a significant role. Disorders such as sleep apnea, restless leg syndrome, and chronic pain can severely impact sleep quality. For instance, sleep apnea causes repeated interruptions in breathing during sleep, leading to fragmented and non-restorative sleep. Addressing these conditions through medical interventions and lifestyle modifications is essential for improving sleep.

Exercise is another critical factor in this interplay. Regular physical activity has been shown to enhance sleep quality by reducing stress and promoting physical tiredness, which can facilitate easier and deeper sleep. However, it's important to time exercise appropriately, as vigorous activity too close to bedtime can increase alertness and body temperature, making it harder to fall asleep. Morning or early afternoon workouts are generally more conducive to promoting better sleep at night.

The Interaction Between Mind, Body, and Sleep

The mind and body do not operate in isolation; they interact continuously, influencing sleep patterns and quality. Psychological stress can manifest in physical symptoms such as muscle tension and elevated heart rate, which can further impede sleep. Conversely, physical discomfort or illness can lead to anxiety and stress, creating a vicious cycle that exacerbates sleep problems.

Creating a harmonious balance between mind and body is key to navigating this landscape. Establishing a consistent sleep routine that aligns with the body's natural circadian rhythm is fundamental. This includes going to bed and waking up at the same times every day, even on weekends. Ensuring the sleep environment is conducive to rest by keeping the bedroom cool, dark, and quiet can also help.

Integrating holistic practices such as yoga, tai chi, and mindfulness can enhance this balance. These practices promote relaxation, reduce stress, and improve physical health, all of which contribute to better sleep. Nutrition also plays a role; a balanced diet rich in nutrients supports overall health and can influence sleep patterns. Avoiding heavy meals, caffeine, and alcohol close to bedtime can prevent disruptions in sleep.

Healing From Within: Revolutionary Strategies For Inner Balance And Sleep Restoration

In today's fast-paced world, the quest for better sleep and inner balance has become more critical than ever. Revolutionary strategies for achieving this involve a holistic approach that considers both mental and physical health. By focusing on inner balance and sleep restoration, we can unlock the potential for profound healing and enhanced well-being.

The Foundation of Inner Balance

Inner balance is the equilibrium between the mind, body, and spirit. Achieving this balance is essential for overall health and optimal sleep. When we are balanced internally, our body systems function harmoniously, leading to better sleep and increased resilience against stress and illness.

1. Mindfulness and Meditation: These practices are at the forefront of strategies to restore inner balance. Mindfulness involves being present in the moment, which can reduce stress and promote relaxation. Meditation goes a step further by helping to quiet the mind, lower cortisol levels, and prepare the body for restful sleep. Regular practice of mindfulness and meditation has been shown to improve sleep quality and duration by calming the nervous system and reducing the impact of stress.

2. Breathwork: Breathwork techniques, such as deep breathing exercises and pranayama, can significantly enhance inner balance and promote sleep restoration. Deep, controlled breathing stimulates the parasympathetic nervous system, which helps to reduce stress and induce a state of relaxation conducive to sleep. Techniques like the 4-7-8 breathing method or diaphragmatic breathing can be practiced before bed to prepare the body for sleep.

Nutritional Strategies for Sleep Restoration

Nutrition plays a crucial role in maintaining inner balance and promoting restorative sleep. The food and drink we consume can either support or hinder our sleep quality.

1. Balanced Diet: A diet rich in whole foods, including fruits, vegetables, lean proteins, and whole grains, provides the necessary nutrients for overall health and optimal sleep. Specific nutrients, such as magnesium, found in leafy greens and nuts, and tryptophan, found in turkey and dairy, are particularly beneficial for sleep. These nutrients support the production of melatonin and serotonin, hormones that regulate sleep.

2. Herbal Supplements: Certain herbs and supplements have been traditionally used to promote sleep and restore balance. Valerian root, chamomile, and lavender are known for their calming effects and can help improve sleep quality. Melatonin supplements can be useful for regulating the sleep-wake cycle, particularly for those with irregular sleep schedules or circadian rhythm disorders.

Physical Activity and Sleep

Regular physical activity is essential for maintaining inner balance and promoting sleep restoration. Exercise reduces stress, improves mood, and helps regulate the sleep-wake cycle.

1. Timing of Exercise: While exercise is beneficial for sleep, timing is crucial. Engaging in vigorous physical activity too close to bedtime can increase alertness and body temperature, making it harder to fall asleep. Morning or early afternoon workouts are generally more conducive to promoting better sleep at night.

2. Types of Exercise: Different forms of exercise can have varying effects on sleep. Aerobic exercises like walking, running, and swimming can improve sleep quality by reducing anxiety and depression. Yoga and tai chi combine physical movement with mindfulness, promoting relaxation and reducing stress, making them excellent choices for improving sleep.

Cognitive Behavioral Strategies

Cognitive Behavioral Therapy for Insomnia (CBT-I) is a revolutionary approach that addresses the psychological and behavioral factors contributing to sleep disturbances. CBT-I helps individuals change negative thoughts and behaviors related to sleep, promoting healthier sleep patterns and restoring inner balance.

1. Sleep Restriction: This technique involves limiting the amount of time spent in bed to match the actual amount of time spent sleeping. Over time, this can help consolidate sleep and reduce nighttime awakenings.

2. Stimulus Control: This strategy aims to strengthen the association between the bed and sleep. It involves going to bed only when sleepy, using the bed only for sleep and sex, and getting out of bed if unable to sleep within 20 minutes.

3. Cognitive Restructuring: This involves identifying and challenging negative thoughts and beliefs about sleep. By replacing these with more positive and realistic thoughts, individuals can reduce anxiety and improve their sleep quality.

Holistic and Integrative Approaches

Integrative approaches combine conventional and alternative therapies to promote inner balance and sleep restoration. These may include:

1. Acupuncture: This traditional Chinese medicine practice involves inserting thin needles into specific points on the body to promote energy flow and restore balance. Acupuncture has been shown to improve sleep quality by reducing stress and promoting relaxation.

2. Aromatherapy: The use of essential oils, such as lavender and chamomile, can promote relaxation and improve sleep. Aromatherapy can be incorporated.

Chapter 4: The Fuel Of Transformation: Nutrition And Sleep Synergy

In the pursuit of optimal health, the interplay between nutrition and sleep often goes underappreciated. However, emerging research underscores the critical synergy between these two factors. Proper nutrition can significantly enhance sleep quality, while adequate sleep can improve metabolic health and dietary choices, creating a virtuous cycle of well-being. Understanding this bidirectional relationship is essential for leveraging nutrition as a powerful tool for sleep transformation.

The Impact of Nutrition on Sleep

1. Macronutrients and Sleep: The balance of macronutrients—carbohydrates, proteins, and fats—in one's diet can profoundly affect sleep patterns. Carbohydrates, particularly complex carbohydrates, can enhance the availability of tryptophan in the brain, a precursor to the sleep-inducing hormone melatonin. Consuming a balanced dinner with whole grains, vegetables, and lean proteins can facilitate a smoother transition into sleep.

2. Micronutrients and Sleep: Micronutrients such as vitamins and minerals are crucial for maintaining sleep health. For instance, magnesium, found in leafy greens, nuts, and seeds, is known for its role in muscle relaxation and promoting deep sleep. Zinc, present in foods like meat, shellfish, and legumes, has been linked to improved sleep onset and quality. Vitamin D, often obtained from sunlight and foods like fatty fish and fortified dairy, plays a role in regulating sleep-wake cycles.

3. Timing of Meals: The timing of food intake is also crucial. Eating large, heavy meals close to bedtime can disrupt sleep due to indigestion and increased metabolic activity. Conversely, a light snack containing complex carbohydrates and protein, such as a banana with peanut butter or a small bowl of oatmeal, can promote sleep by maintaining stable blood sugar levels and increasing serotonin production.

Foods That Promote Sleep

1. Tryptophan-Rich Foods: Foods high in tryptophan, such as turkey, chicken, milk, and bananas, can enhance sleep quality by boosting serotonin and melatonin production. Incorporating these foods into the evening meal or as a pre-bedtime snack can facilitate better sleep.

2. Melatonin-Rich Foods: Certain foods naturally contain melatonin, the hormone that regulates sleep-wake cycles. Tart cherries, grapes, tomatoes, and nuts like almonds and walnuts can help improve sleep quality. A small serving of tart cherry juice before bed, for example, has been shown to increase sleep duration and quality.

3. Magnesium-Rich Foods: As previously mentioned, magnesium is a vital mineral for sleep. Incorporating foods such as spinach, pumpkin seeds, and dark chocolate into your diet can help promote relaxation and deeper sleep.

The Effect of Sleep on Nutrition

1. Sleep and Appetite Regulation: Sleep plays a crucial role in regulating hormones that control appetite.

Insufficient sleep can disrupt the balance of ghrelin (the hunger hormone) and leptin (the satiety hormone), leading to increased hunger and a preference for high-calorie, carbohydrate-rich foods. This imbalance can result in weight gain and a range of metabolic problems.

2. Sleep and Metabolism: Adequate sleep is essential for maintaining a healthy metabolism. Chronic sleep deprivation can impair glucose metabolism and insulin sensitivity, increasing the risk of type 2 diabetes and other metabolic conditions. By ensuring sufficient sleep, the body can more effectively regulate blood sugar levels and overall metabolic health.

3. Cognitive Function and Dietary Choices: Sleep quality affects cognitive functions such as decision-making, impulse control, and emotional regulation, all of which influence dietary choices. Poor sleep can lead to increased cravings for unhealthy foods and reduced willpower to make nutritious choices. Ensuring adequate sleep supports better decision-making and adherence to a healthy diet.

Strategies for Enhancing Nutrition and Sleep Synergy

1. Balanced Diet: Emphasizing a diet rich in whole foods—fruits, vegetables, whole grains, lean proteins, and healthy fats—can support both sleep and overall health. Avoiding excessive sugar, caffeine, and processed foods, particularly in the hours leading up to bedtime, can prevent sleep disruptions.

2. Regular Meal Times: Establishing regular meal times helps regulate the body's internal clock and supports stable blood sugar levels. Consistent eating patterns can prevent late-night hunger and promote a more regular sleep schedule.

3. Hydration: Staying adequately hydrated is essential for sleep health. Dehydration can lead to discomfort and disrupted sleep. However, it's important to balance fluid intake to avoid waking up frequently during the night to use the bathroom.

4. Mindful Eating: Practicing mindful eating can enhance the connection between nutrition and sleep. Being aware of what and when you eat can help you make better food choices and recognize the impact of diet on sleep quality. Techniques such as chewing slowly, savoring flavors, and listening to hunger and fullness cues can promote better digestion and sleep.

Beyond Diet: Nourishing Your Sleep And Energizing Your Days

In the pursuit of holistic health, it's essential to recognize that nutrition alone isn't enough to ensure restful sleep and energized days. A comprehensive approach that integrates lifestyle habits, environmental factors, and stress management is necessary to nourish your sleep and sustain high energy levels. This multifaceted strategy goes beyond diet, focusing on creating a balanced and health-promoting daily routine.

Creating a Sleep-Conducive Environment

The environment in which you sleep plays a critical role in determining the quality of your rest. A sleep-conducive environment can make a significant difference in how well you sleep and how refreshed you feel upon waking.

1. Optimal Bedroom Conditions: Ensuring that your bedroom is cool, quiet, and dark can help improve sleep quality. Consider using blackout curtains to block out light and a white noise machine or earplugs to mask disruptive sounds. Additionally, maintaining a comfortable mattress and pillows suited to your sleeping preferences is crucial for preventing discomfort and sleep disturbances.

2. Minimizing Screen Time: Exposure to screens before bedtime can interfere with the production of melatonin, the hormone that regulates sleep. Blue light emitted by phones, tablets, and computers can trick your brain into thinking it's still daytime, delaying the onset of sleep. To counter this, establish a tech-free wind-down period of at least an hour before bed, allowing your body to naturally transition into sleep mode.

Lifestyle Habits for Better Sleep

Your daily habits and routines have a profound impact on your sleep patterns. Incorporating healthy lifestyle practices can enhance both the quantity and quality of your sleep.

1. Regular Physical Activity: Engaging in regular exercise can help regulate your sleep patterns and improve overall sleep quality. Strive to engage in at least 30 minutes of moderate exercise on most days of the week. However, try to avoid vigorous activity close to bedtime, as it can increase alertness and make it harder to fall asleep.

2. Consistent Sleep Schedule: Maintaining a consistent sleep schedule by going to bed and waking up at the same time every day helps regulate your body's internal clock. This consistency reinforces a healthy sleep-wake cycle, making it easier to fall asleep and wake up naturally.

3. Relaxation Techniques: Incorporating relaxation techniques into your nightly routine can help prepare your mind and body for sleep. Practices such as deep breathing, progressive muscle relaxation, and mindfulness meditation can reduce stress and anxiety, facilitating a smoother transition into sleep.

Stress Management and Emotional Health

Emotional well-being and stress management are integral to achieving restorative sleep and maintaining high energy levels throughout the day. Chronic stress and unmanaged emotions can severely disrupt sleep patterns and deplete energy reserves.

1. Mindfulness and Meditation: Regular mindfulness practice and meditation can help manage stress and improve emotional health. These techniques encourage a state of relaxation and mental clarity, which can reduce nighttime rumination and enhance sleep quality.

2. Cognitive Behavioral Therapy (CBT): For those struggling with chronic insomnia or sleep disorders, Cognitive Behavioral Therapy for Insomnia (CBT-I) is a highly effective treatment. CBT-I addresses the underlying thoughts and behaviors that contribute to sleep problems, promoting healthy sleep habits and improved emotional regulation.

3. Journaling: Keeping a journal can be a therapeutic way to process emotions and reduce stress before bedtime. Writing down your thoughts and worries can help clear your mind, making it easier to relax and fall asleep.

Nutrition and Its Complementary Role

While diet alone isn't the sole factor in nourishing sleep and energizing your days, it still plays a complementary role in this holistic approach.

1. Balanced Nutrition: A diet rich in whole foods, such as fruits, vegetables, whole grains, lean proteins, and healthy fats, supports overall health and can indirectly improve sleep quality. Avoiding excessive caffeine and sugar, especially in the hours leading up to bedtime, helps prevent sleep disruptions.

2. Hydration: Staying adequately hydrated throughout the day is important for overall health, but it's wise to limit fluid intake in the evening to avoid frequent trips to the bathroom during the night.

3. Mindful Eating: Practicing mindful eating helps ensure that you're nourishing your body with the right foods and recognizing how different foods affect your sleep and energy levels. Paying attention to how you feel after eating certain foods can guide better dietary choices that support both sleep and daytime energy.

The Sleep Diet Revolution: Transforming Your Plate, Transforming Your Sleep

In recent years, the concept of the "sleep diet" has gained traction among health enthusiasts and researchers alike. The idea is simple yet revolutionary: by transforming what we eat, we can significantly enhance the quality of our sleep. This approach goes beyond traditional sleep hygiene practices, recognizing the profound impact that nutrition has on our sleep patterns. By carefully selecting and timing our meals, we can create a diet that not only nourishes our bodies but also promotes restful and restorative sleep.

The Connection Between Diet and Sleep

The relationship between diet and sleep is bidirectional. Just as poor nutrition can lead to sleep disturbances, inadequate sleep can affect our dietary choices and metabolism. Understanding this interplay is crucial for leveraging nutrition to improve sleep quality.

1. **Macronutrient Balance:** The balance of carbohydrates, proteins, and fats in our diet can influence how well we sleep. Carbohydrates, particularly complex ones, can help increase the availability of tryptophan, an amino acid that promotes the production of serotonin and melatonin—key hormones in regulating sleep. Including a mix of complex carbohydrates like whole grains, vegetables, and legumes in your evening meal can help facilitate better sleep.

2. **Micronutrient Intake:** Certain vitamins and minerals are essential for sleep health. Magnesium, found in leafy greens, nuts, and seeds, plays a role in muscle relaxation and sleep regulation. Zinc, present in foods

like meat, shellfish, and legumes, supports healthy sleep patterns. Additionally, vitamin B6, found in fish, potatoes, and bananas, helps convert tryptophan to serotonin, further aiding sleep.

3. Timing of Meals: When we eat can be just as important as what we eat. Consuming a heavy meal too close to bedtime can lead to discomfort and indigestion, disrupting sleep. Ideally, dinner should be consumed at least two to three hours before bed, allowing time for digestion. A light snack that includes a mix of protein and carbohydrates, such as a small bowl of oatmeal or a banana with almond butter, can be beneficial if you're hungry before bed.

Foods to Promote Better Sleep

1. Tryptophan-Rich Foods: Foods high in tryptophan, such as turkey, chicken, eggs, and dairy products, can help boost serotonin and melatonin levels, promoting sleepiness. Incorporating these foods into your evening meal or as a bedtime snack can improve sleep onset and quality.

2. Melatonin-Rich Foods: Some foods naturally contain melatonin, the hormone that regulates sleep-wake cycles. Tart cherries, grapes, tomatoes, and nuts like almonds and walnuts are excellent sources. Drinking a small glass of tart cherry juice or having a handful of nuts before bed can enhance sleep.

3. Magnesium-Rich Foods: Magnesium is crucial for muscle relaxation and promoting deeper sleep. Foods such as spinach, pumpkin seeds, and dark chocolate can help ensure adequate magnesium intake. Incorporating these foods into your diet can help alleviate insomnia and improve sleep quality.

4. Herbal Teas: Herbal teas like chamomile, valerian root, and passionflower have been traditionally used to promote relaxation and sleep. Sipping on a warm cup of herbal tea an hour before bed can create a soothing pre-sleep ritual that signals your body it's time to wind down.

Avoiding Sleep Disruptors

1. Caffeine: While caffeine can enhance alertness and performance during the day, consuming it too late can interfere with sleep. It's best to avoid caffeinated beverages and foods at least six hours before bedtime.

2. Alcohol: Although alcohol can initially make you feel sleepy, it disrupts the sleep cycle and reduces the quality of sleep. Limiting alcohol intake, especially close to bedtime, can help maintain better sleep patterns.

3. Sugary Foods and Refined Carbohydrates: High sugar intake and refined carbohydrates can cause blood sugar spikes and crashes, which can disrupt sleep. Choosing whole, unprocessed foods over sugary snacks and desserts can help stabilize blood sugar levels and promote more restful sleep.

Creating a Personalized Sleep Diet

Developing a sleep-friendly diet involves personalizing your food choices and meal timings to suit your unique needs and lifestyle.

1. Listening to Your Body: Pay attention to how different foods affect your sleep. Keep a food and sleep diary to track what you eat and how you sleep each night. This can help identify patterns and foods that either help or hinder your sleep.

2. Gradual Adjustments: Make gradual changes to your diet rather than drastic overhauls. This allows your body to adjust and helps create sustainable habits. Start by incorporating more sleep-promoting foods and gradually reducing intake of sleep disruptors.

3. Consulting Professionals: If you have persistent sleep problems or dietary concerns, consider consulting a healthcare provider or a nutritionist. They can offer personalized advice and develop a plan tailored to your specific needs.

Chapter 4: The Sleep Evolution In Action: Overcoming Challenges, Unlocking Potential

Sleep is a fundamental pillar of health and well-being, yet achieving and maintaining optimal sleep can be challenging for many. The concept of "sleep evolution" emphasizes the need to adapt and refine our approach to sleep in response to modern-day challenges. By understanding and addressing these obstacles, we can unlock our full potential and reap the benefits of restorative sleep.

Understanding Modern Sleep Challenges

In today's fast-paced world, several factors can impede our ability to get quality sleep. These challenges are often multifaceted, involving physical, psychological, and environmental elements.

1. Stress and Anxiety: One of the most significant barriers to good sleep is stress and anxiety. The pressures of work, personal life, and other responsibilities can lead to overactive minds that make it difficult to relax and fall asleep. Chronic stress can also contribute to sleep disorders such as insomnia.

2. Technology and Blue Light Exposure: The ubiquitous presence of screens in our lives has a profound impact on sleep. Blue light emitted by smartphones, tablets, and computers can suppress melatonin production, delaying sleep onset and reducing sleep quality. Late-night screen use can also keep the mind engaged, making it harder to unwind.

3. Irregular Schedules: Shift work, travel across time zones, and inconsistent sleep patterns can disrupt the body's internal clock, leading to difficulties in falling asleep and waking up at regular times. This misalignment can result in a condition known as circadian rhythm disorder.

4. Lifestyle Factors: Poor dietary choices, lack of physical activity, and substance use (such as caffeine, alcohol, and nicotine) can negatively affect sleep. For example, consuming caffeine late in the day can delay sleep onset, while alcohol might help you fall asleep initially but can disrupt sleep later in the night.

Strategies for Overcoming Sleep Challenges

To overcome these challenges and evolve our sleep habits, a proactive and comprehensive approach is necessary. This involves making intentional changes to our routines and environments to support better sleep.

1. **Stress Management Techniques:** Implementing stress reduction strategies can significantly improve sleep quality. Practices such as mindfulness meditation, yoga, deep breathing exercises, and progressive muscle relaxation can help calm the mind and prepare the body for sleep. Additionally, cognitive-behavioral therapy (CBT) has been shown to be effective in treating chronic insomnia by addressing the underlying thought patterns and behaviors that contribute to sleep difficulties.

2. **Creating a Sleep-Conducive Environment:** Optimizing your sleep environment is crucial for overcoming sleep challenges. This includes maintaining a cool, dark, and quiet bedroom. Investing in a comfortable mattress and pillows, using blackout

curtains to block out light, and employing white noise machines or earplugs to mask disruptive sounds can create an ideal setting for sleep.

3. Limiting Screen Time: Reducing exposure to screens before bedtime can help improve sleep quality. Establishing a digital curfew—turning off electronic devices at least an hour before bed—can allow the body to produce melatonin naturally. Instead, engage in relaxing activities such as reading a book, taking a warm bath, or practicing gentle stretching.

4. Regular Sleep Schedule: Maintaining a consistent sleep schedule, even on weekends, can help regulate the body's internal clock. Going to bed and waking up at the same time each day reinforces healthy sleep patterns and makes it easier to fall asleep and wake up naturally.

5. Healthy Lifestyle Choices: Adopting a balanced diet, regular physical activity, and avoiding substances that can interfere with sleep are crucial steps. Eating a light evening meal with sleep-promoting foods, engaging in regular exercise (but not too close to bedtime), and limiting caffeine and alcohol intake can all contribute to better sleep.

Unlocking Your Sleep Potential

By addressing these challenges and implementing effective strategies, we can unlock the full potential of our sleep. Quality sleep has far-reaching benefits, including enhanced cognitive function, improved mood, better physical health, and increased productivity.

1. Enhanced Cognitive Function: Adequate sleep is essential for memory consolidation, problem-solving, and creative thinking. When we sleep well, we perform better academically and professionally, making more effective decisions and retaining information more efficiently.

2. Improved Mood and Emotional Regulation: Sleep plays a critical role in regulating emotions and managing stress. Sufficient rest can lead to a more positive outlook, reduced irritability, and better emotional stability. This, in turn, fosters healthier relationships and a higher quality of life.

3. Better Physical Health: Quality sleep supports aspects of physical health, including immune function, cardiovascular health, and metabolic regulation. It helps repair and rejuvenate tissues, reduces inflammation, and lowers the risk of chronic conditions such as diabetes and heart disease.

4. Increased Productivity: When we are well-rested, we have more energy and focus to tackle daily tasks. This leads to greater efficiency and productivity in both personal and professional endeavors, allowing us to achieve our goals more effectively.

The Power of Persistence: Navigating The Journey To Sleep Evolution

Achieving and maintaining optimal sleep is a journey that requires dedication, patience, and resilience. The power of persistence is crucial as we navigate this path, facing challenges and setbacks along the way. By staying committed to our sleep goals and continuously adapting our strategies, we can ultimately transform our sleep habits and improve our overall well-being.

Understanding the Role of Persistence

Persistence is the quality that allows us to keep moving forward despite difficulties or delays in achieving our goals. When it comes to sleep, persistence means consistently applying and refining sleep hygiene practices, even when progress seems slow or elusive.

1. Setting Realistic Goals: The journey to better sleep starts with setting realistic and achievable goals. This might include gradually adjusting your sleep schedule, improving your sleep environment, or incorporating relaxation techniques into your nightly routine. By setting manageable goals, you create a roadmap that guides your progress and helps maintain motivation.

2. Tracking Progress: Keeping a sleep diary can be an invaluable tool for tracking your progress and identifying patterns. Documenting your sleep habits, the quality of your sleep, and any factors that may have influenced it can provide insights into what works and what doesn't. This information allows you to make informed adjustments to your sleep strategy.

3. Adapting to Challenges: Challenges are inevitable on the journey to better sleep. Whether it's stress, changes in routine, or health issues, it's important to remain flexible and adaptable. Persistence involves recognizing that setbacks are part of the process and using them as opportunities to learn and grow.

Strategies for Maintaining Persistence

1. Developing a Consistent Routine: One of the most effective ways to improve sleep is by establishing a consistent bedtime and wake-up time. This helps regulate your body's internal clock and reinforces healthy sleep patterns. Even if you experience occasional disruptions, returning to your routine as soon as possible can help maintain progress.

2. Creating a Supportive Environment: Surrounding yourself with a supportive environment can enhance your persistence. This includes making your bedroom conducive to sleep, as well as seeking support from family and friends. Sharing your sleep goals with loved ones can provide encouragement and accountability.

3. Prioritizing Sleep: Treating sleep as a non-negotiable priority is essential for persistence. This might mean making sacrifices in other areas of your life, such as limiting late-night social activities or reducing screen time before bed. By prioritizing sleep, you reinforce its importance and create the conditions necessary for success.

Overcoming Common Obstacles

1. Managing Stress and Anxiety: Stress and anxiety are common obstacles to good sleep. Developing effective stress management techniques, such as mindfulness meditation, deep breathing exercises, or cognitive-behavioral therapy, can help reduce their impact on your sleep.

2. Dealing with Irregular Schedules: For those with irregular schedules, such as shift workers or frequent travelers, maintaining a consistent sleep routine can be challenging. Strategies such as light therapy, strategic napping, and creating a dark, quiet sleep environment can help mitigate the effects of irregular schedules.

3. Addressing Sleep Disorders: If you suspect you have a sleep disorder, such as insomnia, sleep apnea, or restless legs syndrome, seeking professional help is crucial. A healthcare provider can diagnose and treat these conditions, helping you achieve better sleep.

The Long-Term Benefits of Persistence

Persisting in your efforts to improve sleep can yield significant long-term benefits. Quality sleep is linked to numerous aspects of physical and mental health, including:

1. Enhanced Cognitive Function: Adequate sleep improves memory, concentration, and problem-solving skills. This can lead to better performance at work or school and a greater capacity for creative thinking.

2. Emotional Well-Being: Good sleep is essential for emotional regulation and resilience. It helps reduce symptoms of anxiety and depression, leading to a more stable and positive mood.

3. Physical Health: Quality sleep supports immune function, cardiovascular health, and metabolic regulation. It reduces the risk of chronic conditions such as obesity, diabetes, and heart disease.

4. Increased Productivity: When well-rested, you have more energy and focus to tackle daily tasks. This leads to greater efficiency and productivity in both personal and professional endeavors.

Chapter 5: Awakening To Your New Reality: Embracing Life Beyond Sleep

Achieving consistent, high-quality sleep is transformative, but the true value of this transformation extends beyond the bedroom. As you awaken to a new reality of improved rest, you also embrace a richer, more vibrant life. This newfound vitality touches every aspect of your existence, from mental clarity and emotional stability to physical health and social interactions. Embracing life beyond sleep means leveraging the benefits of restorative rest to enhance your daily experiences and overall well-being.

Mental Clarity and Cognitive Function

Quality sleep is fundamental to cognitive performance. With adequate rest, you'll notice a significant improvement in mental clarity, memory, and decision-making abilities. This cognitive boost translates into greater efficiency at work or school and a sharper mind for problem-solving and creativity.

1. Enhanced Memory: Sleep plays a crucial role in consolidating memories. During the deeper stages of sleep, your brain processes and stores the information you've acquired throughout the day. This leads to better recall and retention, making learning new skills and absorbing knowledge more effective.

2. Improved Focus: A well-rested mind is more attentive and focused. You'll find it easier to concentrate on tasks, avoid distractions, and maintain a high level of productivity. This enhanced focus can significantly impact your performance and output in professional and personal endeavors.

3. Creative Thinking: Restorative sleep fosters creative thinking and innovation. As your brain sorts through information during sleep, it can make novel connections and generate fresh ideas. This creative edge can benefit various aspects of life, from work projects to personal hobbies.

Emotional Stability and Resilience

Sleep is also crucial for emotional regulation. With consistent, high-quality rest, you'll experience greater emotional stability, resilience, and overall mental health.

1. Mood Enhancement: Adequate sleep helps regulate mood and reduces the risk of mood disorders such as depression and anxiety. You'll wake up feeling more refreshed and positive, ready to tackle the day with a brighter outlook.

2. Stress Reduction: Quality sleep helps mitigate the effects of stress. It enables your body to recover from the day's stresses and prepare for the next. As a result, you'll feel more equipped to handle challenges and less overwhelmed by daily pressures.

3. Emotional Resilience: Well-rested individuals are better able to manage their emotions and respond to situations calmly and rationally. This resilience allows for healthier relationships and more effective conflict resolution, enhancing your social interactions and overall quality of life.

Physical Health and Vitality

The benefits of good sleep extend to your physical health, promoting vitality and longevity. Embracing life beyond sleep involves recognizing and optimizing these physical benefits.

1. Energy Levels: Adequate sleep replenishes your energy stores, leaving you more invigorated and ready to engage in daily activities. You'll find you have more stamina for exercise, work, and leisure activities, enhancing your overall quality of life.

2. Immune Function: Sleep is vital for a robust immune system. It helps your body fight off infections and illnesses, reducing the frequency and severity of sickness. This improved immune function means fewer sick days and a more active, engaged life.

3. Physical Fitness: Quality sleep supports muscle recovery and growth, essential for physical fitness. Whether you're an athlete or just enjoy staying active, good sleep enhances your physical performance and helps prevent injuries.

4. Chronic Disease Prevention: Consistent, restorative sleep reduces the risk of chronic conditions such as obesity, diabetes, and cardiovascular diseases. By prioritizing sleep, you invest in your long-term health and well-being.

Social Connections and Relationships

Restorative sleep also positively influences your social life and relationships. With better sleep, you'll find it easier to connect with others and maintain healthy, fulfilling relationships.

1. Improved Communication: A well-rested mind is more patient and empathetic, enabling better communication and understanding in your interactions. You'll be more present and engaged in conversations, fostering deeper connections with those around you.

2. Enhanced Social Engagement: With more energy and a positive outlook, you'll be more inclined to participate in social activities and engage with your community. This active social life can enrich your experiences and provide a sense of belonging and support.

3. Stronger Relationships: Quality sleep contributes to emotional stability and resilience, which are crucial for maintaining strong, healthy relationships. You'll be better equipped to navigate conflicts and support your loved ones, leading to more harmonious and fulfilling connections.

Personal Growth and Fulfillment

Embracing life beyond sleep involves harnessing the benefits of restorative rest for personal growth and fulfillment. With better sleep, you have the clarity, energy, and resilience to pursue your passions and achieve your goals.

1. Pursuing Passions: Quality sleep provides the mental and physical energy needed to explore and develop your interests. Whether it's learning a new skill, advancing your career, or engaging in creative projects, good sleep supports your endeavors and helps you excel.

2. Achieving Goals: A well-rested mind and body are more capable of setting and achieving goals. You'll find it easier to plan, prioritize, and stay motivated, driving you toward success in various aspects of life.

3. Personal Fulfillment: Ultimately, embracing life beyond sleep means experiencing a deeper sense of fulfillment and joy. With the benefits of restorative sleep, you'll live a more balanced, productive, and satisfying life, fully embracing each moment and opportunity.

The Dawn of Transformation: Harnessing The Potential Of Sleep Evolution

The dawn of transformation through sleep evolution marks a pivotal moment in understanding and optimizing our well-being. This concept revolves around not merely achieving better sleep but fundamentally transforming our lives by harnessing the potential that quality rest offers. By embracing sleep evolution, we unlock a myriad of benefits that touch every facet of our existence, from mental and physical health to emotional resilience and overall life satisfaction.

The Science Behind Sleep Evolution

Sleep is a complex and dynamic process that profoundly affects our health. It consists of multiple stages, each playing a crucial role in our body's recovery and regeneration. Understanding these stages and how they contribute to our well-being is fundamental to harnessing the full potential of sleep evolution.

1. NREM and REM Sleep: Non-Rapid Eye Movement (NREM) sleep has three stages that range from light to deep sleep, each serving distinct purposes like physical restoration and immune system strengthening. Rapid Eye Movement (REM) sleep, on the other hand, is crucial for cognitive functions such as memory consolidation, learning, and emotional regulation. By ensuring a balanced progression through these stages, we maximize the restorative benefits of sleep.

2. Circadian Rhythms: Our internal body clock, or circadian rhythm, regulates sleep-wake cycles and is influenced by external cues such as light and temperature. Aligning our sleep patterns with our natural circadian rhythms enhances sleep quality and overall health. This synchronization allows our body to perform optimally, boosting energy levels, mood, and productivity.

Strategies to Harness Sleep Evolution

1. Creating a Sleep-Conducive Environment: The foundation of sleep evolution lies in optimizing our sleep environment. This includes ensuring a comfortable mattress and pillows, maintaining a cool and dark room, and minimizing noise. Techniques such as using blackout curtains and white noise machines can help create an ideal sleeping sanctuary, promoting uninterrupted rest.

2. Consistency and Routine: Establishing and maintaining a consistent sleep schedule is crucial. Going to bed and waking up at the same time every day, even on weekends, reinforces your body's internal clock. This regularity enhances sleep quality and makes falling asleep and waking up easier.

3. Mind-Body Relaxation Techniques: Incorporating relaxation practices into your nightly routine can significantly improve sleep quality. Techniques such as deep breathing, progressive muscle relaxation, and mindfulness meditation help calm the mind and prepare the body for sleep. These practices reduce stress and anxiety, common barriers to quality sleep.

4. Healthy Lifestyle Choices: Nutrition and physical activity profoundly impact sleep. Consuming a balanced diet rich in sleep-promoting nutrients like magnesium and tryptophan can enhance sleep quality. Regular physical activity, especially aerobic exercise, helps you fall asleep faster and enjoy deeper sleep. However, it's important to avoid vigorous exercise close to bedtime, as it can be stimulating.

5. Limiting Stimulants and Disruptors: Reducing the intake of caffeine and alcohol, particularly in the hours leading up to bedtime, can significantly improve sleep. While alcohol might help you fall asleep initially, it disrupts sleep later in the night. Similarly, limiting exposure to electronic screens before bed helps mitigate blue light's impact on melatonin production, facilitating a more natural sleep onset.

The Transformative Benefits of Sleep Evolution

By committing to sleep evolution, we open the door to a host of transformative benefits that enhance various aspects of our lives.

1. Cognitive Enhancement: Quality sleep improves cognitive functions such as memory, attention, and problem-solving skills. This cognitive boost translates into better performance at work or school and a greater capacity for creative thinking and innovation.

2. Emotional Well-Being: Sleep is vital for emotional regulation. Consistent, quality sleep reduces the risk of mood disorders like depression and anxiety. It enhances emotional resilience, allowing us to navigate stress and challenges more effectively and fostering a more positive outlook on life.

3. Physical Health: Sleep supports numerous aspects of physical health, from boosting immune function to regulating metabolism. Adequate sleep helps reduce the risk of chronic conditions such as heart disease, diabetes, and obesity. It also supports physical performance and recovery, making it essential for athletes and fitness enthusiasts.

4. Social and Interpersonal Relationships: Good sleep enhances our ability to engage and connect with others. Improved mood and emotional stability contribute to healthier and more fulfilling relationships. Being well-rested makes us more patient, empathetic, and better communicators, enriching our social interactions.

5. Overall Life Satisfaction: The cumulative effects of quality sleep enhance our overall life satisfaction. With improved mental and physical health, emotional well-being, and stronger relationships, we can enjoy a more balanced, productive, and fulfilling life. Sleep evolution empowers us to realize our full potential and live life to the fullest.

Living Fully Awake: Embracing Your Transformed Life With Gratitude And Purpose

The journey toward optimal sleep is not merely about resting well; it's about waking up to a transformed life where you can live fully awake. When you achieve consistent, restorative sleep, you unlock a profound shift in how you experience and engage with the world. Living fully awake means embracing this transformation with gratitude and purpose, recognizing the gifts that quality sleep bestows upon your mind, body, and spirit, and channeling this newfound vitality into a life of meaning and fulfillment.

Embracing Gratitude

Gratitude is a powerful mindset that can significantly enhance your quality of life. As you begin to experience the benefits of better sleep, cultivating gratitude can deepen your appreciation for this transformation and its positive impacts.

1. Acknowledging the Benefits: Start by consciously acknowledging the improvements in your life due to better sleep. Notice the increased energy, mental clarity, emotional stability, and overall well-being. Reflect on how these changes enhance your daily experiences and interactions.

2. Practicing Daily Gratitude: Incorporate a daily gratitude practice into your routine. This could be as simple as writing down three things you are grateful for each morning or evening. By focusing on the positive aspects of your life, you reinforce a mindset of thankfulness and contentment.

3. Sharing Gratitude: Expressing gratitude to others can also strengthen your sense of appreciation. Take time to thank those who have supported your journey to better sleep, whether it's family members, friends, or healthcare providers. Sharing your gratitude can deepen your connections and spread positivity.

Living with Purpose

With the mental and physical benefits of quality sleep, you are better equipped to pursue your passions and live a purposeful life. Purpose provides direction and motivation, helping you make meaningful contributions and find satisfaction in your endeavors.

1. Identifying Your Purpose: Reflect on what brings you joy and fulfillment. Consider your values, interests, and talents. What activities make you lose track of time? Identifying your purpose involves understanding what drives you and aligns with your core values.

2. Setting Meaningful Goals: Once you have a clearer sense of purpose, set specific, achievable goals that align with it. These goals should challenge you but also be realistic and attainable. Break them down into smaller, manageable steps to make progress feel more achievable and maintain momentum.

3. Taking Action: Purpose is brought to life through action. Dedicate time each day to work toward your goals, whether it's learning a new skill, volunteering, pursuing a hobby, or advancing your career. Consistent effort and perseverance are key to making your purpose a central part of your life.

Enhancing Relationships

Living fully awake also involves nurturing your relationships. Quality sleep improves your mood and emotional regulation, making you more present and engaged with others. Embrace this transformation to strengthen your social connections and build a supportive community.

1. **Deepening Connections:** Use your enhanced energy and focus to invest in your relationships. Spend quality time with loved ones, actively listen, and show genuine interest in their lives. Deepening these connections can provide emotional support and enrich your social life.

2. **Being Present:** Practice mindfulness to be fully present in your interactions. Put away distractions, such as phones and electronic devices, and focus on the moment. Being present enhances the quality of your

interactions and helps build stronger, more meaningful relationships.

3. Giving Back: Engage in acts of kindness and generosity. Volunteering or helping others not only benefits those around you but also enhances your sense of purpose and fulfillment. Giving back fosters a sense of community and reinforces the positive impacts of your sleep transformation.

Nurturing Your Well-Being

Living fully awake requires ongoing attention to your overall well-being. Continue to prioritize your sleep and incorporate other healthy habits to maintain and enhance your quality of life.

1. Prioritizing Self-Care: Make self-care a regular part of your routine. This includes not only maintaining good sleep hygiene but also engaging in activities that promote relaxation and reduce stress. Practices such as yoga, meditation, and spending time in nature can help maintain balance and well-being.

2. Physical Health: Continue to engage in regular physical activity and maintain a balanced diet. Exercise and nutrition play crucial roles in supporting sleep quality and overall health.

3. Mental Health: Pay attention to your mental and emotional health. Seek support if needed, whether through counseling, support groups, or talking to trusted friends and family. Prioritize activities that bring you joy and satisfaction, and be mindful of your mental well-being.

Conclusion: The Sleep Revolution Continues

As we reach the end of this exploration into the transformative power of sleep, it becomes clear that the journey toward optimal rest and its myriad benefits is an ongoing revolution. The Sleep Revolution is not just a fleeting trend or a temporary fix; it is a fundamental shift in how we understand, prioritize, and harness the power of sleep to enhance our lives. This revolution continues to unfold as scientific research advances, societal attitudes evolve, and individuals commit to embracing healthier sleep practices.

The Science of Sleep: A Continuous Evolution

The scientific community's understanding of sleep has grown exponentially, yet it continues to evolve. Research into the intricate mechanisms of sleep and its impact on health and well-being is constantly revealing new insights. This ongoing discovery process underscores the complexity of sleep and its profound importance.

1. **New Discoveries:** Researchers are continually uncovering new aspects of sleep, such as the roles of different sleep stages, the impact of sleep on various bodily systems, and the connections between sleep and mental health. These discoveries help refine our approach to sleep health, leading to more effective strategies for improving sleep quality.

2. **Technological Advancements:** Innovations in technology are providing new tools for monitoring and enhancing sleep. Wearable devices, sleep apps, and smart home technology offer personalized insights and solutions, making it easier for individuals to understand and improve their sleep patterns.

3. **Public Awareness**: As scientific understanding grows, so does public awareness. Educational initiatives and media coverage are helping to shift societal attitudes toward sleep, highlighting its importance and encouraging healthier sleep behaviors.

Personal Commitment: The Heart of the Revolution

While scientific advancements and societal shifts are crucial, the heart of the Sleep Revolution lies in personal commitment. Each individual's dedication to prioritizing sleep and adopting healthy practices fuels this ongoing movement.

1. Consistency and Persistence: Achieving and maintaining quality sleep requires consistent effort and persistence. Establishing and adhering to a regular sleep schedule, creating a conducive sleep environment, and practicing relaxation techniques are fundamental habits that need to be nurtured over time.

2. Adaptability: Life's circumstances are ever-changing, and so too must be our approach to sleep. Whether it's adjusting to new work schedules, dealing with stress, or managing health conditions, being adaptable and proactive in maintaining good sleep hygiene is essential.

3. Lifelong Learning: The journey toward optimal sleep is a lifelong learning process. Staying informed about new research, experimenting with different strategies, and continuously refining one's sleep routine can help sustain long-term sleep health.

Broader Impacts: Society and Beyond

The Sleep Revolution extends beyond individual benefits, impacting society as a whole. As more people prioritize sleep, the ripple effects can lead to broader societal improvements.

1. Public Health: Improved sleep across populations can lead to better overall public health. Reduced rates of chronic illnesses, enhanced mental health, and lower healthcare costs are just a few of the potential benefits of widespread sleep health.

2. Productivity and Creativity: In workplaces, schools, and other settings, better sleep can enhance productivity, creativity, and innovation. Well-rested individuals are more focused, motivated, and capable of high-level thinking, contributing to more effective and dynamic environments.

3. Community and Relationships: Quality sleep fosters emotional stability and resilience, which are critical for healthy relationships and community engagement. As individuals experience better sleep, their ability to connect, empathize, and collaborate improves, strengthening the social fabric.

The Future of the Sleep Revolution

Looking ahead, the Sleep Revolution holds immense promise. Continued advancements in sleep science, technology, and public awareness will drive further progress. However, the true power of this revolution lies in its collective momentum—the more people who join and commit to prioritizing sleep, the greater the impact.

1. Integrative Approaches: The future of sleep health will likely involve integrative approaches that combine traditional wisdom with modern science. Holistic practices such as mindfulness, yoga, and natural remedies will complement technological and medical advancements, offering comprehensive solutions for sleep health.

2. Global Collaboration: Addressing global sleep challenges requires collaboration across borders and disciplines. Researchers, healthcare providers, policymakers, and communities must work together to create environments that support healthy sleep for all.

3. Sustainable Practices: Sustainable sleep health involves practices that can be maintained over the long term. This includes promoting environments that support natural sleep-wake cycles, encouraging work-life balance, and fostering cultures that value rest and recovery.

The Path Forward: Embracing The Ever-Evolving Landscape Of Sleep And Life

As we delve deeper into the importance of sleep, it becomes evident that the journey towards optimal rest and well-being is a dynamic, ever-evolving process. Embracing this fluidity requires a commitment to continuous learning, adaptation, and proactive management of our sleep habits. The path forward is about recognizing that our sleep needs and circumstances will change throughout our lives, and our approach must evolve accordingly.

Understanding Sleep as a Lifelong Journey

Sleep is not a static state but a dynamic process that changes with age, lifestyle, and health status. This understanding is crucial as it underscores the need for a flexible approach to managing sleep.

1. Life Stages and Sleep Needs: Throughout different stages of life, our sleep requirements and patterns shift. Infants need significantly more sleep than adults, while teenagers often experience shifts in their circadian rhythms that make them prone to staying up later. As we age, sleep quality may decline, necessitating adjustments in our sleep hygiene practices.

2. Health and Sleep: Health conditions, both chronic and acute, can significantly impact sleep. Conditions like sleep apnea, chronic pain, and mental health disorders require specific strategies and sometimes medical intervention to manage effectively. Staying informed about these impacts and seeking appropriate help is crucial for maintaining sleep health.

3. Lifestyle Changes: Major life events, such as starting a new job, moving to a different time zone, or having a child, can disrupt sleep patterns. Understanding how to adapt to these changes while maintaining good sleep hygiene is key to navigating these transitions smoothly.

Continuous Learning and Adaptation

The landscape of sleep science is continually advancing, offering new insights and strategies for improving sleep. Staying engaged with these developments can help you adapt your sleep practices effectively.

1. Stay Informed: Regularly seek out reliable sources of information about sleep health. This could include following scientific publications, health blogs, or attending seminars and workshops focused on sleep.

2. Experiment and Adjust: What works for one person might not work for another. Be open to experimenting with different sleep strategies and routines. Whether it's adjusting your bedtime, trying new relaxation techniques, or modifying your sleep environment, find what works best for you and be willing to adjust as needed.

3. Utilize Technology: Advances in technology have provided us with tools to monitor and improve our sleep. Wearable devices, sleep apps, and smart home devices can offer valuable insights into your sleep patterns and suggest personalized improvements.

Building Resilience Through Sleep

Resilience, the ability to bounce back from stress and adversity, is closely linked to sleep. Prioritizing sleep can enhance your resilience, enabling you to handle life's challenges more effectively.

1. Mind-Body Connection: Recognize the connection between your mental state and sleep. Stress and anxiety can significantly impact sleep quality, so it's important to incorporate stress management techniques into your routine. Practices such as mindfulness, meditation, and deep breathing exercises can promote relaxation and better sleep.

2. Healthy Lifestyle Choices: Regular physical activity, a balanced diet, and avoiding excessive caffeine and alcohol are foundational to good sleep. These choices not only improve sleep but also contribute to overall health and resilience.

3. Social Support: Foster strong social connections, as they can provide emotional support that buffers against stress. Engaging in social activities and maintaining relationships can enhance your sense of well-being and indirectly improve your sleep.

Embracing Change with a Positive Mindset

Embracing the ever-evolving nature of sleep and life requires a positive mindset. Viewing changes as opportunities for growth rather than obstacles can make a significant difference.

1. Flexibility and Openness: Cultivate a flexible attitude towards your sleep practices. Life is full of unexpected changes, and being adaptable can help you maintain good sleep hygiene despite these fluctuations.

2. Growth Mindset: Adopt a growth mindset, seeing challenges in your sleep and health as opportunities to learn and improve.

3. Self-Compassion: Be kind to yourself during this journey. There will be nights when sleep is elusive despite your best efforts. Practicing self-compassion can help reduce the frustration and stress that can further disrupt sleep.